Yoga Fitness Secrets

Lose Weight and Tone Up Body With Yoga Exercises

Tammy Thomas

Copyright

Terms of Use

Any information provided in this book is through the author's interpretation. The author has done strenuous work to reassure the accuracy of this subject. If you wish you attempt any of the practices provided in this book, you are doing so with your own responsibility. The author will not be held accountable for any misinterpretations or misrepresentations of the information provided here.

All information provided is done so with every effort to represent the subject, but does not guarantee that your life will change. The author shall not be held liable for any direct or indirect damages that result from reading this book.

Contents

Why Yoga

If you're thinking why yoga would be beneficial for you, here are two reasons: it makes you feel better and it improves your strength, flexibility, and stamina.

The reason why yoga makes you feel better is because yoga helps you clear out your mind. It doesn't matter how stressed out you are or how many different topics are on your mind at the moment.

When you start doing yoga the most important thing to remember is to clear out your mind. This way, your body can relax as you're performing the different yoga poses.

Yoga also improves your strength, flexibility, and stamina because, in a sense, it is a form of exercise. There are many yoga poses that focuses on flexibility and requires some use of your strength.

Unlike normal workouts, yoga doesn't necessarily work up much of a sweat from your body. However, that doesn't mean that you can't improve your stamina from yoga. The results are the same no matter what type of workout you do.

Also, yoga is known to have many health benefits for your body. For one thing, by doing yoga, you can help lengthen your lifespan. Not to mention that yoga can also help lower the effects of asthma, backaches, depression, headaches, and much more.

These are only the selected few of the benefits of yoga. If you want a more specific list then you'll have to research it up online. Note: the list is pretty long.

Changes

For anyone who don't or does celebrate the New Year, you have made a New Year resolution before. I know you have so don't try to deny it. If you haven't then there is clearly an issue. Anyways, even if you have made a New Year resolution, have you ever fully kept them? I know that most of my friends, and even I, have made New Year resolutions that we couldn't keep. Why can't we keep them? That's probably the same reason was to why you can't keep yours.

For those who don't know what I'm talking about, I'm talking about a lack of motivation. Obviously, if you lack motivation to do something then you will have a hard time accomplishing whatever task you lay out for yourself. What's worse is that you'll eventually grow tired and give up because you'll see that it's no longer worth it to continue. It's not a very good ideology to keep up but it's very common. This is probably because you're setting a difficult goal for yourself. Not that I wouldn't want you to challenge yourself, but you should make one that you can keep.

The same applies for any goal that you chose to set for yourself during anytime of the year. Even if it might not be a New Year resolution, it's still a resolution. Once you've set yourself a goal, it's always best to reach it before giving up.

A good idea to keep in mind is that if you want to change certain behaviors, you need to substitute a new pattern of behaviors into your system. You've probably heard of the saying, "old habits die hard".

Well, make a new habit so you can quickly kill the old one. Yes, that sounds brutal. No, it will not kill you.

Taking a Step

The best way to continue something is to start it because, obviously, if you don't start then you can't continue. It's as simple as that. We also know that starting something is a lot easier than continuing something, especially if it's long term. I know that having to continue something is a difficult thing to do.

There have been times where I had given up some of my goals because it took a long time for me to accomplish them. I'm pretty sure majority of the human population has had the same experience. The key is to stop doing that.

The tricky part with success is that you have to believe that you will succeed. Believe that you can succeed is out of the picture. Scratch it, rip it, or burn that thought out from your head.

When taking the first step into your goal, you have to understand that you will fail if you think that you will fail. It's like climbing a tree.

If you keep thinking that you can't do it because it's too high then you won't be able to because you'll give up after your first fall. However, if you keep thinking that you can, you'll be able to climb up because you worked hard to reach your goal. Sure, you may end up with some bruises here and there but that's what trial and error is. You hurt yourself so your body knows for sure that you won't be repeating what you just did to get that bruise. But seriously though, don't do that.

Basically what I'm trying to say is that if you start a goal thinking that you're going to fail then you are going to fail before you've even started. It doesn't matter if you've already started you're going to fail anyways if you keep thinking like that.

Sometimes, it's good to walk into something not being too optimistic about it but that doesn't mean that you should walk in with a pessimist's point of view. Believing that you will fail is entirely different than actually failing in the long run.

Willpower

Willpower is the reason why you are able to still continue with your goal despite the hardships that you face in the long run. If you don't have the willpower, you don't have the drive to keep going. If you don't have the drive to keep going then you're ultimately going to fail.

Saying and doing are completely different. It's like the saying, "Actions speak louder than words." You can say that you want to do something all you want but if you're never going to set yourself up to do it then it's futile.

It's never good to have to force out the willpower to do something. If you feel that you're completely forcing yourself to do something, I suggest you stop doing it. Pushing and forcing requires a different amount of effort.

If you have to force yourself to do something then it's best to do something new or figure out a way to make it fun for you to do. Willpower can only last for so long when it's taking all your efforts just to keep yourself going.

Yoga Myths

Yes, there are yoga myths. That is to be expected since yoga has been around for a very long time. Not to mention that yoga is often portrayed through a professional rather than a complete beginner.

Keep in mind that there are probably more myths than the ones that I've listed, but these are just the selected few. Though, I doubt there are a lot of yoga myths out there to begin with.

Flexibility:

It's true that most yoga poses does require flexibility. However, that doesn't mean that you have to be flexible when you start out as a beginner. The point of yoga is that it improves your flexibility. Meaning that if you're not flexible then you will be once you're a regular.

I know that some yoga poses seems like you would have to be really flexible to do, but it's possible even without much flexibility. The point is that you will practice. By performing simple poses when you're starting out will help improve your flexibility for harder poses in the long run. With yoga it's all about patience.

Girls only:

No. Yoga is not limited to only females. It's open to all genders. It is true that majority of women do yoga as a form of exercise but that doesn't mean that there aren't any men either. I personally haven't seen many men do yoga, but I have seen a few. However, I am not encouraging the fact that yoga is only for women. It's probably because of this myth that most men would rather stick to their traditional weight lifting and paced jogging.

For all the ladies out there, if there is a guy that you have been bugging to get off his feet and do something productive, now is a perfect opportunity to grab him and take him to a yoga class. If he doesn't want to go then tell him to put on some comfortable clothes and take you "out" for a walk or something. Then you can drag him to class with you. It doesn't matter which method you choose as long as you've succeeded in dragging him with you.

Religious:

You don't have to be religious to do yoga. Though it is true that yoga is linked to Buddhism and Hinduism, yoga has no relations to an actual religion. If you're doing yoga, you're not required to take up any religion nor are you required to be religious. You may adopt a religion in the process if you want, but there will be nothing held against you if you don't. Honestly, you can be an atheist and do yoga.

Meditation

For those of you who don't know what meditation is, meditation is a form of practice that allows an individual to train their mind as well as calm it. Basically, if you're stressed, meditation allows you to become unstressed.

Often time, when most people think of meditation they also think of yoga. That is true because yoga and meditation is equally linked to each other. Yoga is a form of exercise that allows you to relax your body while burning calories while meditation helps relaxes your body and cleans your mind. Usually, when you start to do yoga you would also meditate. Well, that's what most people do. It's not mandatory but it's recommended.

If you think that meditating requires a long amount of time then you're wrong. You can meditate for 5 minutes and still obtain as good an effect as if you were meditating for half an hour. This is because everyone works differently from each other, which is why timing isn't an important factor in meditating. Nevertheless, that doesn't mean that you should expect immediate results when meditating. Results take time, especially if you want good results.

How:

The beauty of meditation is that it can be done at any time of the day. It never hurts to clear your mind and relax your body when you're too tense. There's also no set limit as to how many times you can meditate in a day.

By all means, do it once every hour if you love it so much. Trust me; you'll be able to think better when you meditate at least once a day. Back when I used to meditate, it was something that I was forced into doing because of the school that I went to (it was a weekend school). I was actually quite edgy about wanting to do it because I thought that it would be a waste of time to just sit there in complete silence. Yet, after the third time I meditated, I noticed that I was able to think properly compared to before. My body was less tensed and I wasn't so grumpy all the time as I was before. Anyways, just try meditating sometimes. Not only will you be able to feel a change but you'll also enjoy it.

When you're meditating, make sure that your body is positioned properly. If it's not then you won't be able to feel much of an effect as you should have. One thing to consider before you meditate is your environment.

The point of meditation is that you're surrounded by absolute silence. Well I wouldn't say complete silence that you can hear yourself breathing. I mean silent enough so that you can easily relax yourself without being disturbed by loud noises. Unless if you live in a very busy neighborhood where you're constantly listening to the honking of cars and screaming of your neighbors, you need to pick a new location to do your meditation.

While meditating, you are able to listen to music if it helps you relaxes yourself. Make sure that the music you're listening to isn't something that's played on the normal radio station like hip hop or R&B.

Listen to some calm and gentle music whether it's nature music or a soothing piano melody.

If you've ever seen anyone that has ever meditated then you would know what kind of position they would be in. It might look difficult when you see it, but once you're already in the position, it doesn't feel so bad.

Make sure that you're sitting on ground level when you start. If you need cushion then place a pillow under you but be sure that it isn't big enough to throw you off balance when you're meditating.

Secondly, you should maintain a straight back as you meditate. Do not slouch at all. Doing so will only give you further back problems.

Thirdly, relax your whole body. I'm not saying to just let all of your body die out in one go. Slowly release all the tension around the parts of your body. As you're doing this, stop thinking about whatever you were thinking about and breathe. Taking deep breaths can help you relax tremendously well.

Diet

Moving away from yoga for a moment, let's take a good look at the type of food that we should consider when we decide to go on a diet. Everything about dieting starts in the kitchen so before you can head on to exercising you need to know the proper foods to eat.

Remember, you should never starve yourself whenever you're planning on dieting. That's going to backfire on you and make you gain weight rather than lose it. Not to mention that you're going to start having cravings and hunger that's going to be very difficult for you to cope with. That means that the more you crave the harder it will be for you to resist. Thus, you're going to eventually cave in and eat whatever you want to eat.

Calories are important. Learn to balance the amount of calories you consume per day so you won't have to worry about gaining any excessive weight. A good balance to keep is 1,600 calories per day. You can subtract or add from that amount depending on your metabolism. So if you tend to work out a lot during the day then you would add 100 calories or so to your daily balance.

Never eat any low-fat or fat-free food. Those don't necessarily help you lose weight. On the contrary, you're going to gain weight by eating those types of foods. This is because those types of foods are high in sugar due to its lack of taste. Basically, you're eating sugar rather than a legit meal.

When taking foods into consideration, eat whole grains. They are your best friends, right next to vegetables. If you're a vegetable hater then look up some recipes that you can make with them.

There are a lot of different ways you can cook vegetables to your liking. Take fruits into consideration too. Not only can you eat them but you can blend them into a healthy drink. You would want to avoid processed foods. I'm not stating that you can never eat them ever again once you enter a diet. I'm stating that you should try to minimize the amount of processed foods that you eat if you're planning on staying in a diet.

If you're unsure about how you can tell if a food is processed or not then look at the labeling. If the ingredients contain words that you have never seen before, or that you can't simply pronounce, it's a processed food.

For liquids, drink either tea or water. I would recommend you to just drink water overall. For one thing it's good for you. Another reason is that you can't get fat over water. You can drink as many bottles of water as you want but you won't gain a single pound afterwards.

Though, you might feel bloated with all that water in you so you shouldn't drink so much. Drink about 2-3 bottles of water per day, or 4 if you're that thirsty. If you want to drink juice then you should make your own. It's a waste of money to go out to a shop and buy fruit juice because you can make the same drink in your own home.

It's also a lot healthier if you were to make it fresh since you know for sure that the fruits are clean and haven't been left in the fridge for a few days. Not to mention that there is a lot less sugar put into your juice since you're the one making it. The same applies for slush. If there's fruit included then you can do it at home.

There is always the vegetarian diet. Of course, if you're normally a meat eater, you won't become a vegetarian overnight. Many people nowadays are resorting to becoming a vegetarian for health reasons. Though it's not necessarily required, it's not a bad eating habit to consider. You don't even have to be a vegetarian actually.

You can make yourself a plan stating that you will eat only meat around a certain time of the year while the rests are vegetarian food. Besides, you might like it so much that you'll consider being a full fledge vegetarian. If you've never been to a vegetarian restaurant then you should pay one a visit. You'll be amazed as to what you can eat and how well the taste resembles your favorite foods.

Eating Tips:

For the yoga diet (I'm joking. This works for every diet) you should wash yourself first before eating. If it's early in the morning, it's refreshing to take a quick morning rinse before eating breakfast. It'll keep you feeling clean and refresh until your actual shower. When eating, make sure you sit yourself down before taking the first bite of your food. It's not good to eat while standing up or walking around.

Sit somewhere that you would feel most comfortable and eat your food there. It'll make the food taste better.

Everyday, you should have 3 main meals. Of course, there are cases where you would feel hungry between meals, especially when you're constantly active during the day. You can still have snacks in between meals as long as the snacks aren't junk food. You can have up to 2 snacks a day. When eating a snack, you can have a fruit or a light salad, whichever works best for you.

Also, don't be inconsistent with your meals. If you eat at a particular time on one day, try to continue that routine for the following days. If you don't then your eating schedule will be thrown off course and pretty soon, you'll be either eating too early or too late. If you eat too late then your stomach would take a longer time to digest.

Eat with others. It's always fun to be able to have breakfast, lunch, or dinner with your friends or families. It'll make your meal time seem livelier. Plus, sharing is caring. If you're sharing your food then you wouldn't have to force yourself to eat all your food if you can't finish it. You won't even have to throw it away.

Instead of paying for only yourself, invite someone to eat with you and split the cost between the both of you. You'll waste less money and you'll be just as full without any leftovers. Remember to chew your food carefully when you eat. It'll be easier for your stomach to digest if you do. Plus, the slower you eat the easier it will be for you to be full without eating so much.

Only eat when you're hungry. There's no point in eating if you still feel full. It's great that you like to eat. Food is the greatest thing ever, but you should keep your food consumption to a limit. In addition, if you eat when you're not necessarily hungry then your body will have a hard time digesting the food, if it even gets digested at all.

Equipment/Clothing

When doing yoga, you don't necessarily need anything besides your body. Though, since yoga requires a good amount of ground work depending on which pose you do, some people prefer to have a small portable mat with them.

If you're doing exercises in your own home you won't really need anything. However, if you're doing yoga at a class or somewhere else then you would probably want to consider bringing something like that with you. Even a big towel is fine if that's all you have.

As for clothing, pick whatever you feel most comfortable in doing. I wouldn't recommend wearing jeans or very tight clothing when doing yoga, but if that's what you feel comfortable with then by all means. Usually it's best to wear sweat pants and a t-shirt.

You want to wear something that allows you to move freely around when you're doing yoga, especially since most yoga poses requires you to be flexible with your body.

Yoga Poses

Did you know that there are over 2000 yoga poses? If you were amazed then so was I. Even if I'm writing about yoga right now, in the beginning, I actually did not believe that there was over 2000 poses until I did my research. Though I will not give you all 2000 poses in this book (you'll probably not bother to read it if I did) I have included a couple of poses that you can do on a daily basis, including warm up poses and main poses.

For the main poses, there are different levels of difficultly for each pose so it's fine if you can't do some of them when you're starting out. The point is to be able to master the easy poses first and then move on to the harder poses.

Don't be afraid to work slowly. If it's taking you at least a week to master a pose then that's perfectly fine. Speed is nothing in yoga. You are trying to have a relaxed exercise while burning additional calories. So work at your own pace and do whatever you feel comfortable with. If there's a pose that you feel that you can't do then don't do it. Do other poses and come back to that one on a later date.

Also, if you feel pain when you're doing some of these poses then its best if you stop. If you feel a sudden pain when doing yoga then you're either doing something wrong or you need to have a physical examination with your doctor. This would be common since you'll be stretching and opening muscles that you would never have known that it was there.

Of course, there is good pain too but I'm sure you'll be able to differentiate by which one is which just by the feeling of it. Don't worry if your body starts to sore up. After every new workout it's expected that you will be sore.

Additional information that you need to keep in mind when practicing yoga is that you should practice yoga on an empty stomach. It might sound weird to you but think about it. If you are full when you are practicing yoga then you can end up with stomach pains because the food that you've eaten hasn't fully digested yet. Either that or you can practice an hour or so after you've eaten.

I've probably said this before, but I'll say it again: don't do yoga in an open place. Unless if the place you are at is quiet, calm, relaxing, and there are also other people doing yoga there then you can practice in an open place. Other than that, I suggest practicing in a quiet room. Note that if you do practice outside make sure that you're surrounded by clean air.

In yoga, you'll be breathing a lot so you wouldn't want to be breathing in pollution. Also, don't forget to meditate when you finish. It's always good to end a yoga practice with a deep relaxation of the mind and body.

Keep in mind that you don't have to do the same poses everyday. Switch it around every so often. If you're limited on time then you don't have to do the main poses. Make sure that you do at least do 2-3 basic or warm-up poses per day just to keep your body active. It doesn't have to be in one sitting.

If you don't have time then you can do one pose in the morning and then the rest in the afternoon or at night. Don't try speeding through the poses because you won't be able to get the results that you want. When you do a series of different poses in one sitting, make sure that you take short break intervals in between.

So after you've finished a pose, you should take about a 10-20 second break before moving on to the next pose. This way, it can relieve the tension in your body and relaxes your muscles from the previous pose. When resting, lay your body flat down with your hands placed next to you until your breathing returns to normal. Try not to fall asleep.

Lastly, as you're doing yoga, remember to breathe slowly. If you take quick breaths all the time then you're not going to be able to get much effect from the exercises that you're doing. When doing yoga, you're going to be required to breathe a lot in order to relax your body during those poses. Don't try to cheat and take quick breathes. That's like you wanting to gain muscles but not actually lifting the appropriate weight that you're supposed to. In the end, it's going to be a waste of time. Remember, zero effort is zero progress.

Keep in mind that results do not happen immediately. For some poses, it's expected that you will be able to feel immediate results. However, for the other majority of poses, results will take time. This is why you shouldn't try to cheat when you're doing yoga.

The quicker you skim through these poses the longer it'll take for your body to show results. Take it step by step and take it slowly.

Warm Up

These are a few basic warm-ups that I am providing you with. The good thing about warm-up exercises is that it isn't very difficult to do. Unlike the more advance poses, you won't necessarily be required to be flexible.

In a sense, some of these warm-up poses might even improve your flexibility. None of these are in any particular order so you can just simply pick and perform. Majority of these poses will also help you warm up the spine, shoulder, and hips.

The Long Salutation:

This pose can be difficult in the beginning for some people since it requires pressure on the toes. However, it is a good way to stretch your upper body.

Basically, you start by kneeling down with your palms together and extending your arm upwards. Keep your arms close to your ears and bend forward as if you're bowing down. Make sure that your nose and forehead touches the floor while your butt is touching your heels. Your arms should still be stretching as your body is bent. If you can't keep your arms completely stretched out like you had before then it's ok to bend them a little bit to your needs.

Hold that position for at least 8 seconds and repeat the pose for as many times as you want.

The Yoga Posture:

This pose is known to be a very easy posture. Unfortunately, if you have a lot of weight around your stomach then you'll have a harder time doing this pose since it requires you to bend while sitting. Even so, don't fret over it. Just do the best that you can.

For starters, make sure that your sitting on a flat surface. Cross both of your legs together like Indian style (that's what my teachers called it when I was young). Put both of your hands behind your back and grab a hold of your left wrist with your right hand. From there, bend your body forward until your nose and forehead is nearly touching the floor. If your head isn't touching the floor then that's perfectly fine. I don't believe anyone is able to perform something of that caliber no matter how flexible they may seem to be.

Hold the pose for 8 seconds before pulling your body back up again. Remember, inhale before bending and exhale when bending. Repeat the pose for as many times as you want.

Alternate Elbow/Knee:

This pose is fairly easy. It's an abdominal strengthening exercise that helps strengthens the core, building heat in your body, and waking up the spine.

To start, begin by lying on your back, bringing your knees to a right angle. Be sure to keep your ankles flexed and your toes spread out from each other. Link your fingers together, placing them behind your head and bring your elbows in, keeping them shoulder width apart. Once you're into position, inhale on your back. When you're exhaling, curl your chest up to your thighs. Your thighs should be straight on top of your hips. Maintain that position and inhale once more while extending one of your legs forward. As you're starting to exhale, with the same side that you stretched your leg, twist and lift up your rib cage off the floor. Basically, if you extend your left leg then you would lift up the left side of your rib cage, but if you extend the right leg then you would lift up the right side of your rib cage.

Once you're done, inhale once more, unwind your body, and repeat the process with a different side. Repeat this process as many times as you want. Make sure that you're inhaling and exhaling at the right time.

Cat:

The reason this pose is called the cat pose is because you're required to be on all fours. The reason why the word cat is chosen is due to the next pose which we will talk about later. For this pose you are warming up your spine, opening your hips, and releasing the tension within your shoulders.

When starting, start on your hands and knees. Be sure to line your wrist beneath your shoulders and to keep your knees under your hips. Basically, if you were to draw an imaginary line from your knees to your hips then they should be parallel to each other. Spread out both your fingers and toes and release the weight of your body through your hands, shins, and feet. Inhale while creating a backbend in your spine and you're lifting your chin up. Exhale and start lifting up your back until your spine makes an upward curve. Bring your chin towards your chest as you lift the front of the body up towards the back of the body. Repeat this process as many times as you want.

Cat Balance:

Cat Balance is the more advance version of Cat. In this pose, you're basically balancing your body while you are in a stretched position. This pose helps strengthens your back and your abdomen.

Start on your hands and knees. Your wrist should be parallel to your shoulders and your knees should be parallel to your hips. Basically, you're starting with the basic Cat position. Stretch one of your arms forward and extend the opposite side of your leg. So if you're stretching you're right arm then you're extending the left side of your leg. Maintain that position and hold it for at least 4 breaths. Remember not to breathe too fast. Return to your original position and repeat the same steps but with opposite sides. Repeat this pose as many times as you want.

Table:

This pose is a little bit more difficult than the previous poses, but its good practice for strengthening your back posture as well as your shoulders and arms. This pose is quite useful for those with stiff necks or those who has had neck injuries.

To begin, sit down and place your hands behind you. Bend your knees and position your ankles until they are parallel to your knees. As you're inhaling, lift your hips, low back, and thighs off of the floor. It might be difficult on the first time but if you keep practicing then you'll be able to do it easily. Make sure that you're comfortable in that position. If you're not then you shouldn't try remaining in the pose because there might be a chance that you can hurt yourself. However, if you're easily able to perform that pose then hold the position for 4 breaths. If your neck is perfectly fine then throw your head back while you're in the position. Repeat this pose as many times as you want.

Table Balance:

Table Balance is the harder form of Table. I would only recommend that you move onto this pose only after you've completely mastered the table pose. Table Balance is a pose that requires the strength throughout your core and shoulders.

To start, get into table position. Once you're set, extend one of your legs forward and flex out your foot. Hold that position for 4 breaths. When you want to return into the basic position, exhale as you're releasing your leg back down. When you want to switch legs, inhale as you're extending your other leg up. Repeat this process as many times as you want.

Puppy:

This pose is an entry level for the next pose that I will go over called Downward Facing Dog. This pose is supposed to open up your chest, shoulders, and spine.

First, start on all fours. If you pretend that you're an actually puppy it might be really cute. Anyways, stretch out your arms and hands forward like a puppy stretching after waking up. Make sure that your hips are parallel to your knees and start stretching your torso forward. Once you've felt like you've stretched a good amount, come back on all fours.

Simple, right? Repeat this step as many times as you want.

Downward Facing Dog:

This is quite the interesting, but complex pose. It's a harder form of Puppy. It's going to be useful for a later pose so you'll have to do it eventually. Even so, it's not a pose that will be hard for you to master. You can probably get it right on your first time. This pose equally stretches and strengthens your body so I would actually recommend doing this pose first thing in the morning just to warm up your body for the day.

Like Puppy, start on all fours. Then, start to walk on your hands. Take about 2-3 steps forward, not too small and not too big. Once you're done, lift up your hips. Position yourself to make an upside down V. It doesn't have to be perfect. It's fine if you can't stretch that far.

Easy, isn't it? Repeat this step as many times as you want.

Down Dog Kick Back:

This pose is also easy, but it'll require some balance. You can also call this Downward Facing Dog level 2 since the base pose is practically the same.

Start in Downward Facing Dog position. Lift one of your legs up and keep it straight. Hold that pose for as long as you want. Exhale to release and return on all fours and inhale to switch leg. Repeat this step as many times as you want.

Plank:

Before starting, know that this is not the same thing as planking. Those two terms are completely different from each other. For this pose, it helps strengthens your shoulders, arms, and your entire core.

When starting, go into the basic Cat position where you're on all fours. Be sure that your wrist is placed under your shoulders and straighten out your body. Slowly push up and hold that position for 4-6 breaths or until your body cannot hold it anymore. Release and go back on all fours.

This pose is not like doing push-ups. It might be similar but you're trying to hold your body up for as long as you can. You can repeat this pose as many times as you want but make sure that you keep an equal balance of breaths with each push and go slowly.

Side Plank:

This is the more difficult version of the Plank pose. There are actually 2 versions of Side Plank. This just happens to be the easier version. Just like Plank, Side Plank is also good for balance, but it's mainly for the development of side balance. This pose would be helpful for anyone who has had shoulder injuries or have difficulty keeping balance.

Begin by starting out on all fours. Once in position, switch your body to your right hand, knee, and shin. You can start with your left hand, knee, and shin if you prefer that side better. Let's say you're on the right side of your body. Stretch out your left leg and line it up with your right toes. Then open your chest up with your left hand on you hip. You may have trouble balancing but that's alright. If you're balance is perfectly steady then stretch out your left arm up towards the sky or ceiling if you're inside.

Keep that position for a short while and come back on all fours to repeat the other side. Be sure to balance out the amount of time that you take on each side. Repeat this step as many times as you want.

Side Plank Variation:

This is the second version of Side Plank. This version is actually harder than the first version so I suppose you can say that it's a level 3 sort of pose. Don't try to master this pose on the first time if you can't do it. Just practice it one step at a time. Unlike the first Side Plank, this version requires more you to use more of your strength.

To start, go into Downward Facing Dog position. If you know how the pose looks like, you're basically making an upside down V with your body. In simpler terms, start on all fours and lift your hips up. Pick whatever side you want to start with. Let's say we're starting on the right side of the body. So spin onto your right hand and the outer edge of your right foot. Bring your left hand to your hips. Lift up your hips to as high as you can, but don't force yourself to do it. Open up your chest and lift your low back up. This may be a little harder for you to do since your only support system is your hand. Yet, if you can still maintain balance then take your hand away from your hip and raise it up. Hold that position for a while before going back on all fours to repeat the other side. Balance the amount of time that you take on each side. Repeat this step as many times as you want.

Standing

Now you're getting into actual yoga and away from the warm-up poses. Standing poses are the basics of yoga. I highly recommend you master some of these poses first before moving on to other poses that requires a lot of balance. In standing poses, you're mostly on your feet compared to warm-up poses. It helps you bring stability to your lower body. There are probably more standing poses out there but I'm going to list the selected few.

Also, standing poses are very useful for your body because it helps increase stamina, strength, and balance. Even if more of the poses require a different action with both of your legs, it's useful for bringing awareness to your own strengths and weaknesses. These poses will also help strengthen your core. Your hips will become more flexible and your hamstrings will lengthen. After a while, you might even start to feel lighter throughout your lower body. Just keep practicing and exercising.

Mountain:

This is the most foundational pose. This might come off as a very basic pose but it's a pose that you would have to do in order to continue to other poses. Think of it as the first step of everything. If you can't take the first step then you can't go on to the second step. No, hopping does not count.

Basically, in this pose, you're standing on your own two feet. That's it. Yes, anyone can stand but pay attention.

This pose is to strengthen your legs, and abdomen. Even if you're standing on two legs, it also teaches balance. How? Because you're standing still without trying to move.

When starting, stand with your feet together, or if you're feeling stiff then stand with your feet slightly apart from each other. Keep your chin slightly pointed downward and your arms hanging on one side. Rock your body back and forth on the balls of your feet and heels to spread your weight evenly on both feet. Then spread your toes out to give yourself a solid footing. Slightly bend your knees and straighten them again to help you loosen your joints. Curl your pelvic bone up slightly to ensure that your tailbone continues the line of your spine. Extend your spine upward by lifting your chest away from your stomach. Lengthen the back of your neck and relax your throat. Line up your ears directly on top of your shoulders. Finally, press down on the floor with your feet and rest in this position.

Stay in this position for at least 3 breaths before moving on.

Mountain Variation:

There isn't much of a change between Mountain and Mountain Variation. You're basically only moving one body part.

Anyways, start this pose in Mountain position. Raise your arm forward and up over your head. Make sure that your palms are facing each other and that your arms and hands are shoulder width apart. Start to spread open your fingers and strongly breathe out before releasing the pose. So how do you feel?

Runner's Lunge:

This pose activates your leg and gluteal muscles as well as teaches your body balance at the same time. It also increases your strength and endurance.

To start, stand with your feet hip width apart. Step one of your feet back and bring your remaining foot towards a right angle. Basically, if you're starting with your left foot back then you're bringing your right knee toward a right angle. Leave your hands rested on your hips and stay to your center. Try not to move away from the spot that you were standing on before. When you release, straighten your right leg and step the left foot forward. Repeat this step using the opposite side. You can repeat this pose as many times as you want.

Runner's Lunge Variation:

This pose is the same as Runner's Lunge with only a slight change to the pose. It also stretches your shoulders and continues to help develop your lower leg strength.

Start by getting into Runner's Lunge position. Once you're there, sweep your arms forward and up with the palms of your hands facing each other. Your arms and hands should be shoulder width apart.

Repeat this process like how you would in Runner's Lunge but adding in the additional steps in this pose. You can repeat this process as many times as you want.

Runner's Lunge with Twist:

This is another version of Runner's Lunge but with a twist. Unlike the original, this pose requires you to have a good amount of balance and flexibility before you begin. It is supposed to help better your digestion, balance, and mental fortitude. There's another version of this pose but this is the easier one.

To begin, take a long step forward with one of your leg. Bend the front knee of that leg and keep your back leg straight. Whichever leg you start with, use the opposite arm. So if you used your left leg then use your right arm and the same for the other one. Let's say you started with your left leg. Place your right hand on the floor under your left shoulder and keep our right arm straight as you twist your navel, rib cage, and heart toward your left leg. Then, stretch your left arm up and lengthen your spine as you inhale, twisting deeper on exhale.

Return back standing and repeat on the other side of your body. Repeat this process as many times as you want.

Runner's Lunge with Twist Variation:

This is the harder version of the previous pose. It requires more intense balance and posture than the previous one.

To start, start with the Mountain pose. Take a step back with your right foot and bend your front knee to a right angle. Then reach your arms over your head and twist your body. Tuck your right elbow outside your left thigh. Bend your elbows and bring your palms together in front of your chest as if you were praying. Press you right elbow into your left thigh to deepen the twist. Keep your legs steady and stretch through your back heel.

To release this position, exhale. Repeat this process as many times as you want with a different side of your body.

Warrior 2:

This pose is to help strengthen all of your leg muscles and is a fairly easy pose to do.

Begin opening your feet into a wide straddle. Bring your left foot out to a 90 degrees angle and bring your right foot in. Put your hands on your hips and sink your hips down while lifting your chest up. Line the center of your left knee over the center of your left foot. You back leg should stay straight as you're in this position.

Hold this position for 8-10 breaths before releasing. When releasing, straighten both of your legs. Repeat this process as many times as you want with a different side.

Warrior 2 Variation:

This pose is like the previous only with the extension of arms.

Use the same method as you did for Warrior 2 as a base. However, instead of having your hands on your hips, inhale and stretch your arms out to the side, keeping them shoulder height. Relax your shoulder and lift your chest up.

Hold this position for about 8-10 breaths. Repeat this pose like how you would do in Warrior 2 and repeat it as many times as you want.

Bent Knee Triangle:

This pose strengthens the legs and core of your body as well as stretching the spine, the sides of the torso and the shoulders.

Step your feet out into a wide straddle position like how the Warrior pose was. Make sure that your right toes is facing front and your left toes are turned diagonal. Place your hands on your hips and bend your right knee to a right angle. Rest your right forearm on your right thigh and stretch your left arm into the air. Slightly twist your arm and open your chest toward the sky. Straighten your bottom arm, making sure that your finger tips are off the floor and stretch out both arms.

Repeat this process on the other side of your body and repeat it as many times as you want.

Pyramid:

This is a balancing type of pose. It opens your hips and bends your body forward, releasing your lower back.

Start by standing with your feet hip width apart. Set your left foot back 3 steps and keep your toes facing forward with both legs straight. Fold forward your body and place your hands on your kneecaps. Hold this position for about 8-10 breaths before continuing on.

Then, place your hands on your hips, stand up, and step forward. Step your right foot back about 3 feet and keep your toes facing forward and your legs straight. Hinge at the hips and place your hands on your kneecaps. Hold this position for another 8-10 breaths. Finally, take your hands back to your hips, stand up, and step forward.

Repeat this step as many times as you want.

Chair:

This pose is a type of back bend to help strengthen your spine.

Start by standing with your feet hip width apart. Keep your knees bending straight forward as if you were sitting on an invisible chair. Place your hands on your hips then lift your chest up and drop your hips. Make sure that you keep a neutral curve in your spine. Relax your shoulders and hold this position for about 8-10 breaths or to however long you can keep your body up.

Standing Balance

Now that you're done with the basic standing poses, you're now ready to move on to the standing balance poses. It's practically the same only that you're required to have a better sense of balance with these poses since you're mostly going to be standing on one leg rather than two. Make sure that whatever leg that you're using to support yourself with is always going to be straight unless stated otherwise.

Also, these balancing poses will help strengthen your standing leg as well as your core. Of course, your balance will not be consistent. There will be some days where you'll feel more balanced than another. That is also perfectly fine. Eventually, you'll start getting the hang of it and you'll be able to do it consistently.

Toe Balance:

Toe Balance is the beginning pose of this section. Unlike Mountain, which teaches you how to stand, Toe Balance teaches you how to stand and balance from your core muscles by activating your legs. If you have poor balance, don't be afraid to fall. If you're unsure then have something to help your balance as you're going the exercise. Hold onto a chair or a table or something that won't be easily moved.

To start, stand with your feet hip width apart. Keep your hands on your hips and lift up your left leg. If you need help balancing then place the very tip of your left toe on the floor as a guide. Once you're comfortable, slowly start to lift up your toe off the floor.

Hold that position for about 8 breaths before switching.

Knee to Chest:

This pose is similar to Toe Balance except for the fact that you're required to lift your whole leg up. So if you have trouble with toe balance I would recommend that you skip over this and come back later.

To begin, stand with your feet hip width apart. Lift up your left leg and keep your right knee straight while holding onto your left kneecap or shin.

Hold this position for about 8 breaths. Try not to move or lean in any direction. If you feel that your body is starting to become unbalanced then go back on two legs. Don't try to push yourself to stay up. Try to record the amount of time you took to stay up so you can see your improvement when you redo the pose next time. Remember to switch legs after you're done.

Tree:

This pose is to help you maintain your balance on one leg. It's a fairly easy pose and shouldn't be as difficult as you would think it would be.

To start this pose, stand with your feet hip width apart. Bend your left knee and turn your thigh out, placing your left foot on your right inner leg, which is slightly above the ankle. If you're having trouble maintaining your balance then you can place your toes on the floor for stability but it's recommended that you don't.

Try to hold this pose for 8 breaths or for as long as you can. The longer you can hold this position the better your balance will be. Also, when you feel that your balance is improving, try raising your leg up higher on your standing leg. Maintain the time of how long you're balancing on each leg.

Crow:

This pose is a type of arm balancing pose that helps strengthens your upper body. It's a more advance pose than the previous poses so don't be discourage if you can't do it on your first try. It'll probably take you a lot of practice to be able to maintain this pose so don't fret over it.

To start, crouch down to a squatting position. Place your hands shoulder width apart and bend your elbows. Then place your shins on your upper arms and press your shin down into your arms. Tuck your tailbone under and lift your belly up towards your spine. Round up your back and press into your arms with your legs and slowly support yourself up. If you're new to this position then slowly lift one foot up at a time instead of all at once. It'll be useful and safer, especially if you might fall from it. Remember to tuck your heels up toward your body when you're up on the air.

Try to hold your position for as long as you can. Take note of how long you can stay up each time so you can see your progress each time to do this pose.

Spinal Twist

These types of poses would require you to lie on your back rather than to stand. In one way, they can be seem as easy since you're exercise consists of staying on the floor but it's also hard because you're required to bend your body. If you have a low back sensitivity it's recommended for you to go see a doctor or a physical therapist before starting these poses. You can never be too sure. Even then, do not try to force the twist. If you can't do it then hold it off until a later date. In yoga, you're trying to improve your health not to make it worse.

These poses will also help you in your digestion. This is because they increase circulation and movement to your abdominal organs and muscles. They also strengthen your belly and spine.

Double Knee Bend Twist:

The floor is a great place for learning how to twist our body. That's because it helps stabilizes your hips, thus, moving the twists mainly to the spine. Not only that but your abdominal organs gets cleaned out and your spine is made to be more flexible than before. This pose will also open up your chest and shoulders as well as help improve your poster.

To start, lie on your back with your knees at a right angle. Your arms should be at shoulder height as you're maintaining the back of your right shoulders to the floor.

Lower your legs to the left and allow your navel to move with your leg. Stay in this position for at least 4-6 breaths before switching sides. When you inhale, return to the center. For exhaling, turn to the other side.

Straight Leg Twist:

There's actually a lot of work that's to be done in this pose. It's recommended that you work carefully and slowly while you're doing this, especially if you have low back pain.

To start, lie on your back with both knees to your chest. Straighten out your right leg and place the sole of your left foot on top of your right thigh. Then take your right hand to your left knee and twist your left knee across your body and to the right. Make sure that you keep the back of your left shoulder to the floor. Spin your navel to the left and away from the floor and stay in position for about 8 breaths.

Inhale to unwind your body and bring both of your knees back to your chest in order to change sides. Repeat this process as many times as you want.

Back Extension

For these next set of poses you're mainly working on your belly rather than the other parts of your body. If your low back is sensitive then I suggest that you roll up a towel or a small mat under you and place it at the rim of your pelvis. If, in the end, it doesn't help sooth your pain then come back to this section at a later date. I recommend reviewing and mastering the standing pose before heading on to this section since they will help strengthen your core and back.

The Cobra:

This pose is pretty simple but requires you to use your upper body strength. Even if this is a yoga pose you've probably done this pose before when you were in elementary or middle school. At least, that's when I first did it.

Anyways, to start the cobra, start by lying on your chest. Make sure that you're on a flat surface like your floor. If you don't want to hurt your chest then place a mat underneath. Keep your arms rested next to your body. Once you're in position, start supporting your weight on the palms of your hand and slowly raise your chest up, directing your head backwards. There's no specific height that you have to reach so just reach as high as you can. Make sure that you're breathing in while you're raising your body.

Once you've reached the height that you're comfortable with, hold your breath for 8 seconds and breathe out as you're returning to your original position. Repeat this process as many times as you want.

Cobra Variation 1:

There are actually two variations for this pose. Though there's a slight change between both poses, the effects are quite similar. All variations of Cobra focus on the opening of the chest and shoulders as well as the strengthening of the low back and the stretching of the front body.

To begin, lie down on your belly and stretch your arms back, interlacing your fingers together. Squeeze your shoulder blades together and lift your arms away from your torso. Once you're in a comfortable position then start lifting your torso off the ground. Try to hold this position for about 2-3 breaths.

To release, slowly lower your body down and rest one ear to the ground. Lie in one place and relax before moving on.

Cobra Variation 2:

This variation is an intense spinal strengthener as well as strengthens the shoulders.

To begin, lie on your belly and reach your arms forward with your palms facing each other. Inhale and lift your torso and your arms up. Try to level your arms to your ears if you can. Lift your navel towards your spine. Try to hold this position for about 2-3 breaths if you can.

To release, slowly lower your body and rest one ear to the ground. Lie in one place and relax before moving on.

Bridge:

The foundation for this pose is within your feet, outer arms, shoulders, and head. Those parts are crucial in this pose because it provides stability to your body as you're attempting to build a bridge. It is useful for when you would have to lift up your body and support the arching of your spine.

Before starting, lie on your back and bend you knees. Start drawing your heels into your body and take your arms to your side. Once you're in position, lift your hips up in a diagonal line with your knees and shoulders. Press down on the floor with your feet, outer arms, and head. If you feel any pain during this process then stop and rest a bit before coming back to it. If you're fine then start rolling your shoulders under your body and interlace your fingers together. Put more pressure down on the floor through your feet and arms. Then press your low back up and release your navel down. Draw your shoulder blades into your chest, expanding it, and release your shoulders. Hold this position for a short while before releasing.

To release, slowly come down by stretching your arms over your head and lifting your heels. Gently and carefully roll down one vertebra at a time with your tailbone slouching down last.

Wheel:

The Wheel is useful for releasing tension throughout the spine, shoulders, and hips. Note that this pose does not lead up to immediate results but takes time for the effects to appear. It's not an easy pose but rather an intense pose that needs a lot of attention and respect to complete successfully. This pose helps cultivates strength, stamina, and full body flexibility.

To start, lie on your back with your knees bent and your heels drawn towards your body. Bend your elbows and place your hands under your shoulders. Lift up to the top of your head. Keep your elbows about shoulder width apart and equally stand on your hands and feet as you slowly lift your body up. If this is your first time doing this pose then don't move too quickly. You need to go slowly in the case if your body starts to experience any side pains as you're performing this pose. Your arms and legs are your friends in this pose so use them equally as you bend your spine towards a half circular shape. Keep adding pressure to the floor as you try and maintain this pose.

Be very careful when releasing your body. Tuck in your chin to your chest first before bending your elbows. Slowly lower your body down to the ground and rest for a short while before continuing other poses.

Finishing Pose:

Aren't you happy? You're almost done. These next set of poses are called the finishing poses simply because they bring your body back to its neutral state. It's recommended that you do at least 1 or 2 of these poses before you end your yoga exercises. This is because it prepares your body to release any last bit of tension in your hips, pelvis, and low back. Unlike the previous poses, the finishing poses are easy to do and quick to finish.

Hamstring Opener:

To begin, start on all fours. Stretch and straighten your right leg backward and flex your right ankle while pulling your toes back. Keep this position for as long as you want.

Release and switch sides. Make sure that you keep a balance between the amount of time that you spend on each side. Repeat this process as many times as you want.

Hip Opener:

This is a relaxing type of pose so you'll have a very easy time doing this. It's good for stretching out your gluteal muscles and for releasing tension in your lower back.

To begin, lie on your back and bend your knees. Place your left ankle across your right thigh and press your left knee away from your body.

Hold it for a few short breaths before releasing. Repeat this on the other side. Easy right? Repeat this process as many times as you want.

Corpse:

The irony about this pose is that it's not only the easiest pose in this whole book but it's also the hardest. Why? It's easy because all you're expected to do is to lie down and close up your mind. It's hard because you're expected to still your mind.

Basically, when doing this pose, keep your body completely flat on the floor. You can keep your arms and legs together or you can keep them apart from each other. It doesn't matter so just pick whichever position that you're comfortable with. From there, relax every part of your body from head to toe. Start off from your toes first and make your way up. It might sound easy but it's not. If you think you've got it on your first time then you probably didn't. As you're relaxing your body, make sure that your relax everything. You know that you're doing something right if you're trying hard to not let yourself fall asleep. Don't be discouraged if you can't do it after a while. It's probably going to take you a very long time to get it right so don't sweat over it.

Once you feel as if you've relaxed enough, take a few deep breaths and stretch your arms over your head. Bend your knees and roll on to your side. Sit up when you're ready. Take one last breath as you're standing up.

That's it. You're good to go. So how do you feel?

Tracking

Now that you know how to do some of these yoga poses, mix and match them whenever you practice yoga. If there's a pose that you like and you feel that it helps your body then you can continue to do that pose but switch around the rest.

Even so, remember to switch to a new pose after at most 5 weeks. This is because your body will start to get used to the exercise that you're doing and it won't have much of an effect if you're going to continue doing it. That's why it's so good to mix and match, especially if you exercise on a daily basis.

It might seem weird to you but even in yoga you have to keep track of your progress, or at least of what you're doing. I don't care how good you think your memory is. If your memory is good then that's good for you, but you never know when you can forget. I know people whose brains are like computers. They remember everything, which makes me jealous sometimes, but even they can forget the simplest details. I'm not saying that you shouldn't trust yourself. I'm saying that you should record what you do to be on the safe side.

Plus, once you've tracked them, they're stored for life. Well, that's until something happens to it, or it mysteriously disappears. Anyways, it's good to have your data stored for future purposes, especially when you're trying to lose weight.

It's going to be very simple too. You can even write which poses you did for a particular day so when you start changing up your poses you would know which one you did and which one you haven't done.

If you change poses, I would recommend you changing only when you have mastered the pose that you have been working on before. It's not worth changing poses when you haven't even mastered at least one.

You can even be creative with your tracking process. So after you've finished your yoga exercise for the day and you're recording what you've done, leave a space to put a rating right next to each pose.

Basically, you're rating yourself as to how well you did on that pose. I would highly recommend this method because you'll be able to see how well you do on each pose. Remembering which poses you did for the day is one thing but remembering how well you did them is another. Plus, it'll be fun.

You'll be able to clearly see your progress every time you record your data. When recording, chose whatever method you feel comfortable with.

Some people can chose to be simple and put a number ranging from 1-10 with 1 being the worst and 10 being the best. You can also rate yourself by just adding your own comments. An example would be you writing how well or how bad you did on a pose. So let's say that you're recording your progress for the cobra pose.

So if your progress was bad then you would write "need to stay up for 4 more seconds" or something like that. If your progress was good then you would write "held position for all 8 seconds and desired height was reached" or something like that. Do it however you feel comfortable with.

Also, correct yourself. When tracking your progress, don't be afraid to write down something that you did wrong. No one is going to see the journal but you, unless if you show it to other people. However, showing it to other people is entirely up to you.

Regardless, if you feel uncomfortable sharing actual facts with other people in the first place then you shouldn't be sharing. Anyways, if there was something that you did wrong during a certain pose then make sure that you record it. Think of it as a side note for you to remember so you won't repeat the same mistakes twice. You won't improve if you can't remember what to improve on.

Be Active

Though yoga is a good way to exercise, it isn't the only workout that you should do. Even when doing intense yoga, having additional exercises can help your body lose weight. Of course, that doesn't mean that you're going to be losing a lot of weight within a shorter amount of time.

By having additional exercises when you're not doing yoga allows your body to be active even when you're not trying to workout. That doesn't mean that you should go out and lift weights or run a marathon. Just do some simple exercises that will keep you on your feet and of your couch.

Consider walking. Walking is a great way to keep your body active. Yes, walking is also included as a form of exercise. Though you might think that it won't do much by just walking, you would be amaze when you see that your body is burning off some excessive calories.

It's always good to walk about 3 miles per day, which is about 10,000 feet but it's still fine as long as you walk about one mile. It's not very difficult.

If you're planning on driving somewhere that takes about 15 minutes to arrive to then just walk there. It's not a far distance. Of course, the amount of time that it'll take to get there will double but you're receiving exercise at the same time.

Even a 30 minute walk per day is fine. Just walk whenever transportation is not required or necessary. You can even walk to work if you wanted to.

Use the public transportation bus and you'll be saving a lot of gas money.

Here's another idea: community service work. If you're stuck and don't know what to do during your free time, walk around your neighborhood and help out. People are always in need and will be grateful for an extra pair of helping hands. You can even replace exercise with community service work, especially if the work you're doing requires a lot of muscle strength.

In addition, by doing community service work you are helping the community around you. It'll make you feel better at the end of the day when you know that you've done something good for someone else. It'll be a momentary release from your own problems.

There's also the habit of doing your own housework. If you live alone then here's a great opportunity to freshen up your household skills if you haven't already so.

For instance, if you have a habit of ordering take out food most of the times then start learning how to cook. For one thing, eating out isn't very healthy. It doesn't matter if you order take out from a vegetarian place, it's still unhealthy.

This is because when restaurants make their food, it's always loaded with oil and I really doubt that they use new oil after every meal they cook. I would know. I've worked in a restaurant before.

Conclusion

Overall, I would actually recommend that you take up yoga simply because it's a fun way to exercise. It relaxes the tension in your body, improves your flexibility, and trains your muscles.

In addition to that, you're also able to burn off additional calories while you're at it. Don't forget that you should also meditate at least once per day to relax and empty out your mind. Also, the kitchen is your best friend. Learn to love it and learn to use it.

Be sure to keep eating healthy. Whatever you burn off is going to be a waste if the food you're eating isn't letting it stay off. Remember to track your progress and to take up additional exercises whenever you're free and have nothing to do.

Keep eating healthy and try to practice your yoga poses whenever you can. Take it one step at a time.